Slow Down
Ch*by*oice
or Lay Down
by Force

Slow Down *by* Choice *or* Lay Down *by* Force

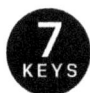

7 KEYS TO RESTORE WHOLISTIC BALANCE IN YOUR LIFE

TRINA PITTS-KHALFANI, BCND, M.Ed.

publish your gift

*This book is dedicated to my two beautiful daughters,
Akilah and Hadiyah, who I strive to teach to be spiritual,
intelligent, courageous young women who exude beauty
inside and out and to always reach for the sky.
If You Can Believe It, You Can Achieve It!*

*Also to my mother, Gloria Jo Scott,
who taught me unconditional love,
who is a caregiver to all, even more than herself.*

TABLE OF CONTENTS

ACKNOWLEDGMENTS

I wish to acknowledge the numerous holistic practitioners and programs that contributed to my education and development along my journey, also, the clients' stories in this book and others who allowed me to learn from their experiences over the years.

I want to particularly thank the few African American holistic practitioners who took the time to teach me in various classes and trainings and from whom I learned a great deal in this field:

Daisy Hawkins, ND, in Harrisburg, PA, who was the first practitioner who took me under her wing and introduced me to this field in my early twenties. Also, Dr. Deidre Burrell and Dr. Wallace Young on the South Side of Chicago, who allowed me to dig even further into alternative holistic health which I attribute to my continuous studies and work in complementary health.

PREFACE

There are periods in our lives when we must just *slow down* and take a pause for our own mental, physical and spiritual health. Our current society tells us that if we are not in constant motion, then we are not striving, not being productive, or lack ambition. Unfortunately, this constant fast-paced lifestyle, which starts at a young age, along with our growing disconnect from the natural resources of the planet, has created a negative impact on our overall health.

As we have become less and less connected to our inner guide and the signals from our bodies, which give us warnings to slow down or realign ourselves back to balance, we then become forced at times to pay attention through physical and/or mental breakdown which results in dis-ease (spelled with a hyphen to emphasize a lack of ease, not the body's normal state). The stories in this book represent real examples of everyday people who needed to be forced to listen to their bodies and slow down in order to renew, regenerate and restore physically, mentally and spiritually.

In *Slow Down by Choice or Lay Down by Force* I will provide you seven keys to help you restore balance and wholeness in your life through examples of my own personal experience and that of clients of how to incorporate basic daily practices that keep you in tune with yourself.

Sometimes in life, we just need to *slow down*!

Trina Pitts-Khalfani, BCND, M.Ed, CNHP
Holistic Practitioner

"Slow Down" by India.Arie

"Slow down baby,
You're going too fast.
You got your hands in the air,
With your feet on the gas.
You're 'bout to wreck your future,
Running from your past.
You need to slow down baby.
Thinking the faster that I go,
The faster that I will reach my goal.
The race is not given to the swift,
But to the one who endureth."

"You can have it all. Just not all at once."
—Oprah Winfrey

Introduction: (Re)awakening

Have you ever felt your heart race so fast that it woke you up abruptly out of a deep sleep so you could catch your breath? And the more you tried to breathe, the faster your heart continued to beat until you felt as if it was going to jump out of your chest and you were going to pass out.

Then begins a cycle of sleepless nights, fatigue, foggy thinking and irritability during the day due to sleepless, anxiety-filled nights. Your appetite goes away, but in comes acid reflux and digestion problems, nervousness with fear-induced anxiety of being alone due to the fear of heart palpitations/heart attack that became more frequent to the point you barely could function.

No health provider could find any medical condition even after being rushed in an ambulance in the middle of the night several times and a four-day hospital stay with a home heart monitor. Multiple doctor appointments and still no definitive diagnosis.

This experience happened to a healthy thirty-seven-year-old married professional mother of a five-year-old and one-year-old. She thought she was doing all the right things, so she did not *choose* to *slow down* and was ultimately *forced* to *lay down* like so many others.

I Am That Woman! That Woman Was Me!

The subtle *yellow* warning lights to *slow down* that I ignored turned to a glaring loud *red stop* light that caught my full attention during the busiest time of my life. There was nothing I could do but *surrender* to the process of creating a more balanced life.

I have always been a go-getter who followed the typical recommended path for the "Modern Woman" who charts her own course in life.

You know:

- Get good grades, successfully finish high school (Class President), and go to college
- Meet your spouse
- Obtain a degree, then a graduate degree
- Get married, and have a big wedding
- Build your career, and buy a home
- Stay fit, have children, then lose the baby weight
- Be a perfect mother
- Start a business, but continue your education
- Join organizations, a religious community and have a social life
- Travel the world
- Give back your time and resources in community service, volunteering at your children's school and extracurricular activities
- Support your spouse and extended family
- And the list just goes on and on.

Whew! I'm getting tired just writing all the things that are supposed to happen based on today's before-the-age-of-forty standards. We are told to pretty much be superwoman with our bedazzled cape who "brings home the bacon" (turkey or vegan bacon please), fries it up in the pan (air fryer) and stays sexy for their man (or another woman will). That's what we are taught to be as Whitney beautifully sang, "I'm every woman. It's ALL in me."

This also applies to men in a different form of expectations and responsibilities all at the same time, with the result being high blood pressure, heart attacks, strokes or worse: premature death.

But the one thing we are never taught to practice is that it is equally important to *slow down* and have periods of *pause* in between all these responsibilities, commitments and expectations so that we can regenerate, revive and renew our mind, body and spirit. Unfortunately I and others had to learn by *force* and not by *choice*, but for me it turned out to be the scariest and most enlightening experience of my life.

My shift and awakening began in 2005 when I just had my second daughter at the age of thirty-five. I also had a four-year-old preschooler. Even though I had my first child at thirty-one, and was at the border of the high-risk stage for pregnancy at my age, I had wanted and needed to space my children apart for my own mental health since I had been a stay-at-home-mother for two and half years with my oldest and just gotten back into my professional career. I didn't marry until twenty-eight after pursuing my bachelor's and master's degrees and starting my career in public health so I waited to become a mother until after the age of thirty when I completed my education and started my career. I became a mother later in my life as I knew that when you have children at a younger age you may have other competing challenges (economics, building your education, career, etc.) that requires another type of juggling act to maintain balance.

Once married, I moved from a small city in Pennsylvania to the big city-living of Chicago, which I felt fit with my various interests and my desire for a fast-paced lifestyle. I quickly became acclimated in a new family and became a socialite, meeting all new people from all walks of life by becoming actively involved in educational, professional and political activities, community grassroots activism, fundraising and faith-based activities while being a new wife, and then becoming a mother after three years. So, for most women including myself, these are the busiest times in our lives and if we are honest, we find ourselves struggling to balance all of these competing responsibilities. Giving each the proper time and attention as well as giving it to ourselves can be a challenge.

I took a period of pause from my professional career after my first child by staying at home for two and a half years and starting my own home-based jewelry and health education consulting business. Once I started back to work, I became pregnant with my second child within a year and worked until the day before my delivery: having contractions at work, literally shopping for my hospital overnight bag hours before delivery and still active in many activities even though I was physically and mentally tired from the pregnancy and managing my life and family.

(Subtle yellow light!)

Since I stayed home for two and a half years and breastfed for six months with my first child, I was determined to go back to work in three months the second time as to not have another interruption in my professional career.

I rushed back in three months, still breastfeeding, constantly rushing, distracted on the job, forgetting things, not getting enough sleep, etc., and after a year of being on autopilot still attempting to do it *all* at the same time, I was awakened abruptly out of my sleep in a cold sweat one night and couldn't breathe.

(Glaring red light. *Literally* . . .)

"There are two causes to suffering: one is forgetfulness, the second is unwillingness."

—Dr. Johnnie Coleman, founding minister,
Christ Universal Temple

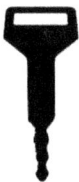

Key 1. (Re)sist

(To oppose actively; fight, argue, or work against, refuse to cooperate with, submit to)

After running from doctor to doctor who just wanted to give me prescriptions for my many symptoms, and after reading about my symptoms in everything I could find to try to self-diagnose, I finally spoke to a cardiologist colleague for her honest opinion and she could not find any medical diagnosis on numerous tests. She finally took off her Medical Provider hat and had a woman to woman (i.e., Sistah to Sistah) talk with me.

"What I want you to do is take two weeks off to de-stress. I'm going to write you a doctor's note and give you bed rest for two weeks," she said.

"Two weeks?! Doing nothing?" I asked. "I have a busy life with two children."

(Re)sisting

She was frank with me: "How are you going to be around for your children if you don't take care of yourself?" (Put your own oxygen mask on first—my first lesson into self-care.)

My cardiologist colleague was emphatic that "everyone would still be fine in two weeks" and wanted to see if it would help.

I trusted her, and since I was living on fumes anyway, I agreed and started with a two-week break, and got the full support of my family. My mother took off and flew from out of town to assist me with the children. I used that time to rest and rejuvenate as much as I could with two children, read everything I could about my symptoms and started to go back to the basics by seeking out various holistic and spiritual practitioners for guidance. At first it seemed like it was getting better as I took time to focus more on my own well-being. After weeks I went back to work and my fast-paced life and then back came the heart palpitations, anxiety and sleepless nights, along now with acid reflux; and then I realized that something else was trying to get my attention. I needed to fully relax, so that I could hear what God was trying to tell me.

As long as I was in motion, I couldn't figure it out. I was too busy breastfeeding, juggling meetings, trying to beat Chicago traffic to get to the daycare before it closed and taking care of the home while at the same time having sleepless nights with tired days with more of the same cycle the next day. I finally surrendered and gave my two weeks' notice and decided to put *me* first and started my journey to wholeness!

Most of us if we are honest have some form of resistance that holds us back or causes us to hesitate or question when presented with new and unfamiliar information, experiences and circumstances. We are creatures of habit and are conditioned to be more comfortable with the familiar belief systems that are passed down from our families, cultures and environments. We ignore symptoms and warning signs and just keep moving because that is what we are taught and accustomed to doing every day. We just keep getting up and doing what we believe we are required to do to survive. But are we really thriving?

We forget in our technologically advanced world, in all our doing and busyness that keeps us disconnected from ourselves, how powerfully and wonderfully we are made in the image and likeness of God and our connection to all of creation in the Universe.

Our bodies have sixty trillion cells with eighty million blood cells that die every second and miraculously the same number are born; we have ten major organ systems that work in conjunction with one another, 630 muscles, and 206 bones. Our heart pumps thirty million times per year with 250,000 gallons of blood over a lifetime. Blood flows through our entire bodies in less than two minutes. We receive new blood every ninety days.

The brain weighs only three pounds but is the computer system (thinking process) of our bodies. Science says light travels at 186,000 miles per second and sound 1,120 feet per second. Spiritual scientists state that "Thought" is the most powerful energy that exists at 24 billion miles per second. And there are also seven chakras (energy centers) that connect the physical with the spiritual aspects of our body.

These facts are an important reminder of the intelligence of our mind, body and spirit to renew itself if given the proper environment/conditions to operate as it was created. We suffer because we forget or never knew this information and we run constantly outside of ourselves for answers to these life-saving truths.

Other times we suffer because we are *unwilling* to listen and do what is necessary to create the balance that we seek in our lives.

When introduced to something new or different, whether it is food, people, activities or even physical, mental or spiritual concepts/ideas, we tend to dismiss it without fully investigating whether it's valuable or can be beneficial to our lives. This shows up as imbalance at times when we are going against the flow or vibrational energy, which sometimes is called your *intuition* (in-tune-to), or the still, small voice/inner spirit that alerts, guides and advises us if we are still enough to listen. When we are constantly in motion the loudness of the external world overpowers that innate wisdom within all of us and we then become disconnected from this powerful resource. This also pertains to the body and dis-ease. When we don't get the message with the warning yellow lights to pause and slow down so that we can hear what it is that we need to be in alignment with our wholeness, then after a period of time of struggling and going against the flow eventually *you* will be *forced* to listen.

Karriem is a relatively healthy forty-year-old male who had pain in his legs as a first sign, which ended up being blood clots. After treatment and testing it was determined he also only had a 30 percent heart function with no other symptoms and no previous heart or health conditions. He struggled and made small attempts over a ten-year period to manage his deteriorating conditions (high blood pressure, heart arrythmias which resulted in a defibrillator, medications, a mini stroke, and weakened kidneys) which deemed him disabled by medical standards. In light of all of these health challenges he still miraculously worked every day (which was surprising to his medical providers); to complicate matters, he also had multiple competing responsibilities (raising children, financial obligations, managing staff as well as running a small business) that created a stressful fast-paced life, even though he was warned to slow down but felt he had to meet all his responsibilities and did not have the luxury of slowing down. In addition to the health challenges he also had multiple emotional traumatic experiences (several unexpected deaths of family members) which led to a constant broken heart and disappointment (heart chakra) which caused a worsening of health challenges (mind-body-spirit connection).

By age fifty-one, Karriem could no longer sustain his health and was required to have a heart transplant with severe life-threatening complications. He was forced to lie down (literally for six months in a hospital) with multiple near-death experiences, and is now by choice attempting to live a stress-free, medically coordinated/controlled life to maintain health which is still a struggle due to his conditioning on how to think and live based on his past experiences and programmed teachings.

Choosing to live differently and incorporating new information is sometimes uncomfortable or scary for us and goes against what we have been taught or conditioned to do by our families or society. You can't act if you don't have correct information but when presented we must be willing to receive it and then act upon it even if it is different than what we are accustomed to in our lives. It can literally be a matter of life or death and also the quality of the remainder of life.

I always use this story that I was told years ago about doing the same things over and over again automatically without questioning whether or not it is working for us:

A wife was cooking Thanksgiving dinner for her family and she cut the turkey in half and cooked each side separately as her young daughter watched with confusion. She asked, "Why are you cooking the turkey that way" and the mother stated, "I don't know, that's how your grandmother taught me." She then called her mother and asked why she taught her that way and the grandmother stated, "That's how my mother taught me." The grandmother then called her mother and asked why she cooked her turkey that way and the great grandmother stated, "Because back in my time the oven was two times smaller than it is today so I had to cook a large turkey a half at a time; I'm not sure why you all are still cooking that way today."

Moral of the story, we need to question whether what we are still doing is necessary and beneficial to our lives.

We have to *remember* the infinite wisdom that is within us all and the universe and be *willing* to hear and listen so we can reconnect with it to create wholeness in our lives.

"Listen to your body talk before it has to scream."

—Unknown

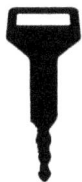

🔑 Key 2. (Re)lax

(Less tense or anxious/rest/make less tight/ To take rest or recreation as from work or effort)

I had to relax and get quiet to better understand why I was having heart palpitations with no heart condition and other debilitating symptoms at the age of thirty-seven even though my tests were all normal. The signs were shown to me and I couldn't ignore them but I kept moving, not acting on them. So, in their own way, my symptoms forced me to stop moving and listen to what they had to tell me.

I started to seek spiritual counseling and take several classes on meditation/relaxation, reading inspirational and self-help books that focus on the mind-body-spirit connection. I had already started in my twenties some holistic practices (colonics, herbs/vitamins, detoxing, etc.) so I was confused why I was having these challenges.

I am a very energetic person who never really knew how to naturally relax so this was all new to me. I thought relaxing was if you could sleep on a good night for about five to six hours. Since I still felt like I was in my prime, sleep was secondary to all the things I needed to get done in a day. And when you are also breastfeeding, well, that is every two to four hours at best that you need to be available to your child. At this point I had given up breastfeeding but still could not get a restful sleep; I had insomnia, (which is a conflict between the mind in arousal state and relaxation).

So basically, you are "wired but tired" and can't calm the mind and get into a state of full complete sleep where the body repairs, rejuvenates and restores itself.

Insomnia is the most common of all sleep disorders. According to the Sleep Foundation, "estimates show that 10% to 30% of adults live with chronic insomnia. For other studies, this figure is closer to 50% to 60%."[i]

According to the Mayo Clinic, "Insomnia is a common sleep disorder that can make it hard to fall asleep, hard to stay asleep, or cause you to wake up too early and not be able to get back to sleep. You may still feel tired when you wake up. Insomnia can sap not only your energy level and mood but also your health, work performance and quality of life."[ii] (Bingo!)

Stress can create hormonal imbalance along with other factors which many women experience as they transition through the perimenopausal (sometimes ten to fifteen years before the menopause stage) of life or after childbirth.

And many Americans, men and women suffer from adrenal fatigue with our high-stress, fast-paced lifestyles which can create low adrenal function. The adrenal glands (referred to as stress glands) are located on top of your kidneys. Though small, they're powerful. They produce essential hormones such as cortisol, which helps you respond to stress amongst other things. When the adrenal glands are imbalanced, they either make too much or not enough hormones.

James Wilson, ND, states in his book *Adrenal Fatigue: The 21st Century Stress Syndrome* "Low adrenal function can create insomnia, depression, hypoglycemia [low blood sugar], chronic fatigue, recurring infections, anxiety, glandular problems and a host of other imbalances in the body."[iii]

With all the stressful experiences that individuals have to navigate daily it is no wonder Americans are experiencing chronic uncontrolled dis-ease (heart attacks, strokes, diabetes, auto-immune disorders, etc.) We are having physical and emotional disorders that impact our ability to *relax*!

One of the best ways I found to relax the mind/body and to de-stress is the practice of meditation. Of course, exercise is also a form of de-stressing for many people; but meditation is slowly becoming popular today as a practice for many of us who were never taught this relaxation technique even though many cultures around the world have utilized meditation for centuries in their daily practice for better health and wellness.

Meditation is the practice of thinking deeply or focusing one's mind for a period of time with deep breathing techniques. This can be done in silence or chanting with music or guided by someone speaking you through the process. It should be done in a sitting position with deep breaths to relax your mind and body without being in a state of sleep. Some of the benefits individuals state are sharper mental function, reduced anxiety, better sleep patterns, increased creativity and spiritual connection.

Deep breathing during meditation is called "the natural tranquilizer!"

Deep breaths:

- Increase serotonin levels and calm the mind
- Allow you to take in more oxygen
- Help eliminate toxins in the lungs
- Lower heart and respiratory rates and blood pressure
- Enhances mood

Sometimes we all just need to take a moment to take a deep breath!

*Khalil is a thirty-nine-year-old male who was running constantly in all areas in life, never taking time to **slow down by choice** before the next goal. He had a full, busy life, moving from one activity to the next every day including weekends. He was an experienced marathon runner, family man, successful professional, multiple business owner and a committed spiritual/community activist. Due to his hectic schedule he didn't have time to properly prepare and hydrate for his next annual marathon. During his run, he collapsed before the finish line, was rushed to the hospital unconscious, and hospitalized for a week with heat exhaustion, severely dehydrated with temporary kidney failure. It took him months to recover. After recovery he continued with his fast-paced lifestyle and had multiple torn meniscus surgeries which required periods of pause and interrupted movement which **forced** him to pace himself and to balance his priorities and responsibilities.*

When you continue to move so fast through life and never take the time to *slow down*, the body/mind will find a way to *force* it upon you and it can be at the most inconvenient, unexpected time in your life. You may think you have it all and life is going as you planned and so, once you reach one goal, you quickly create another and never take time to reflect and restore yourself before the next activity. Even in all the scriptural teachings of creation there was a period of *rest*!

Genesis 2:2 (NIV) says, "By the seventh day God had finished the work he had been doing; so, on the seventh day he rested from all his work."iv

If God the father/mother of all can have periods to relax and rest, then so should the children!

*"Every human being is the author
of his own health or disease."*

—Attributed to Buddha

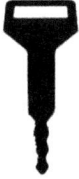

Key 3. (Re)search

(Detailed study into a specific problem
to answer a question)

Since we have entered the Information Age in the late twentieth century, we have at our fingertips (literally) an overwhelming amount of information at our disposal on any topic of interest. It has been a blessing and a downside due to the fact that there is also a large amount of misinformation that can cause confusion about what is truth or just opinion.

We have our cell phones, laptops, tablets, etc. that keeps us on constant overload, where in an instant we can Google or watch a YouTube video or go on social media for all our information any time of the day or night instead of the previous form of research through books, libraries and actual experts in their fields.

When I had my issues, which I found out later were caused by a hormonal imbalance, and I could not find the answer from the medical professionals that I sought out, after feeling confused, frustrated and exhausted, I decided to do my own research and go back to the basics of seeking out information that I learned in college and various self-improvement classes. At first it was overwhelming, as you find so much information that you start to self-diagnose and become even more fearful that you are going to die or have every disease imaginable based on your symptoms. This can be paralyzing as you become more and more afraid (or *resist*) the information which can create a worst-case scenario in your mind which your body then responds to by having even more symptoms (a *psychosomatic* response, which Oxford Languages defines as "a physical illness or other condition caused or aggravated by a mental factor such as internal conflict or stress").[v] It goes back to the famous saying, by Rhonda Byrne from the book *The Secret*, "what you think about you bring about. Your whole life is a manifestation of the thoughts that go on in your head"[vi] (Mind-Body Connection). This is the downside of doing independent research from unverified sources.

The positive side is that when you are determined to find a solution to your issue or health problem, you will leave no stone unturned in your quest for an answer. No one is going to spend as much time as *you* or knows your body the way you do even with all of their medical education/training.

Once I was able to start to relax and get quiet, I was able to listen to my internal guiding (some call it Intuition, God speaking to them or an Epiphany). I believe through my own experience and the experiences of others I have worked with that you will be presented with the right people, information and guided to the right solution for yourself. That requires inner work and no one can do that for you but *you*! Others can guide you, educate you and offer assistance, but healing the mind, body and spirit still requires participation and collaboration on your part and is an inside job.

After running from provider to provider with a hospital stay and numerous tests, I still did not have a definitive diagnosis that I could treat or cure, yet the symptoms still persisted.

I had the benefit and blessing to stay at home and figure it out, which others do not have and have to keep doing their regular routine while trying to heal and manage their dis-eases. Through my journey to balance and wholeness there are a few things that I tried that work for me and that I recommend as a Holistic Practitioner to others. What I always disclose to clients is that everything doesn't work for everybody. There is a buffet of many options and you can choose to select the ones that resonate with you and leave for others the options that they choose to select. Everything that we are learning here is recycled information, and a lot of it has been used in previous times and generations. We have discarded as "antiquated" or "out-of-date" what others are benefitting from around the world and in other cultures. In America we have relied more on modern medical advancements and have forgotten (a cause of suffering) or been unwilling to incorporate techniques, remedies and practices that have stood the test of time and are still beneficial today.

I was in such a desperate state to find answers for my imbalance and dis-ease in my body which was starting to affect my mind and spirit; I was open to almost anything to find relief and get back to a normal way of living. I didn't realize at the time that what I thought was "normal" living was what actually caused me to not be in balance. But most of what we learn today about health and wholeness from our families and pass on from generation to generation is not always the healthiest for us.

I had to relearn and go back to the basics!

BACK TO BASICS

Once I decided to go back to the basics and that my symptoms were not just in my mind and I was not a hypochondriac (someone constantly obsessed about their health) as some tried to have me believe, I tried many alternative therapies before I found what worked for me.

HOLISTIC/ALTERNATIVE/COMPLEMENTARY MEDICINE

According to WebMD, "Holistic medicine is a **form of healing** that considers the whole person—body, mind, spirit and emotions—in the quest for optimal health and wellness. According to the holistic medicine philosophy, one can achieve optimal health—the primary goal of holistic medicine practice—by gaining proper balance in life."[vii]

Holistic practice utilizes a wide range of therapies such as dietary modifications, nutritional supplementation, detoxification processes, acupuncture, chiropractic adjustments, essential oils, spiritual practices (meditation, yoga, prayer), etc.

The basic philosophy is to:

- Do no Harm
- Recognize the healing power of nature

- Identify underlying causes/source of dis-ease and not just treat symptoms
- Involve the total person
- Teach rather than just treat
- Prevent dis-eases

I first was introduced to alternative holistic health in my twenties by a naturopathic doctor named Daisy Hawkins who had a small office on the side of her home in Pennsylvania. She had a large Amish population of clients and I was one of the youngest who would be in her workshops. Dr. Hawkins taught us that "death starts in the colon" due to toxins building in the body and that most Americans are consuming a SAD (standard American diet), in which they lack nutrients and do not have proper frequent eliminations (multiple daily bowel movements), which builds up toxins and inflammation in the body.

In other words, our bodies are poisoning themselves through improper elimination. The information was new to me as a recent college graduate but it seemed practical and interesting. Dr. Hawkins also performed colonics (cleaning of the larger bowel through water irrigation similar to a deep enema). Individuals traveled from all over to receive colonics and her herbal/vitamin recommendations for health. I received my first colonic and started taking vitamins regularly even though I did not have any conditions at the time which she thought it was great for me to start at a young age to prevent illness in the future. That was my first education on disease prevention vs. only disease treatment/management. I subsequently took many young people and family members to her clinic and we traveled together for trainings and workshops as she became my first mentor in Alternative Health.

Many times we have the information but when life happens and we are pulled into multiple roles and responsibilities in our quest for success, money, status and the so-called American dream, we sometimes forget what we know and revert back to the familiar popular route and replace the basics with the next innovative fast-paced, modern way of living at the expense of our mental, physical and spiritual health and well-being.

CHINESE HERBAL MEDICINE

The medical definition of Oriental (traditional) medicine according to Dr. William Shiel Jr. is: "Traditional Chinese medicine (TCM), or Chinese medicine, is an ancient medical system that takes a deep understanding of the laws and patterns of nature and applies them to the human body. TCM encompasses many different practices and is rooted in the ancient philosophy of Taoism which dates back more than 5,000 years."[viii]

Chinese medicine treatments include various forms of herbal medicine, acupuncture, cupping therapy, massage, etc.

I had my first visit with a Chinese medicine practitioner at an office in Chinatown in Chicago. The doctor had traditional Chinese herbs, roots and teas and many clients from a variety of cultures would visit her at her office. She looked at my tongue, took my pulse, had me fill out a health questionnaire and told me I had a cold constitution and a yang deficiency which creates hormonal imbalances. She then proceeded to create a concoction of rocks, herbs, twigs and other items I didn't recognize and told me to boil it twice a day, drain and drink like a hot tea. It looked like a glass of dirt and tasted like it as well. But I tried it and it seemed to calm and relax me. I went a few more times and decided to take a different route but still use various aspects like detox teas and Chinese herbal supplements in my health regime even today as I found it eliminates toxins and assists in balancing the body.

JUICE FASTING/DETOXING/ALKALINE WATER

Fasting is a practice that extends back to biblical times.

Esther 4:16 (NIV) says ,"Go, gather together all the Jews who are in Susa, and fast for me. Do not eat or drink for three days, night or day. I and my attendants will fast as you do."[ix] Matthew 4:1-2 (NIV) says, "Then Jesus was led by the Spirit into the wilderness to be tempted by the devil. After fasting forty days and forty nights, he was hungry."[x]

According to ScienceBlogs.com and a published journal paper in *Physiology*, "animals periodically undergo periods of food deprivation such as during hibernation, mating, molting and migration."[xi]

In nature, individuals fast for many reasons (health, illness, spiritual). Simply put, fasting is primarily a rest from food to allow the body to do what it was designed to do, to regenerate, rejuvenate and repair. For some fasts you do not consume food and others you give up certain foods or activities.

As I continued my research, I found a seventy-five-year-old naturopathic doctor on the South Side of Chicago named Dr. Young. His name was so fitting as he had glowing skin, a youthful energy (ran five miles a day), was a vegan and would sometimes only eat one meal a day. I attended his classes and made an appointment for an evaluation, after which he confirmed my body was out of balance and needed some rest and rejuvenation. He recommended a thirty-day vegetable and fruit juice fast to detoxify my whole body with some herbal supplements to cleanse and build my body. At this point the only reference I had for juice-only fasting for better health was in reading health books in college that discussed this topic like *How to Eat to Live* by Elijah Muhammed and *Heal Thyself* by Queen Afua and other similar books.

Since I was still young and carefree, I had only attempted small health recommendations into my lifestyle. I still didn't believe I could fast on a juice-only diet since I had only fasted a few times before for a few days during Lent (Christian practice) or in solidarity for Ramadan (Islamic practice) but never for that long without any whole foods. Dr. Young convinced me by asking me "has anything else worked for you" and I had to admit it had not fully up to this point.

Dr. Young then educated me that many of us in America have an acidic pH from our acid-forming diets and introduced me to alkaline water. At that point, two of my symptoms were digestion problems and acid reflux which prevented me from eating certain foods like tomatoes, sour apples, etc. or it would burn like crazy in my chest. That was in 2005 and now alkaline water is promoted and sold in many health and grocery stores today. Clients from all over Chicago would bring their empty water containers and pay for his alkaline water that he made in his home office from a water filtration system.

I completed my thirty-day juice fast and detoxed with herbal supplements and consumed alkaline water and I lost thirty pounds and felt great. My skin was glowing and I had an abundance of energy. I was starting to feel normal even though it was initially a struggle; I believe it benefitted me tremendously to reset my body. I then became a student of many of Dr. Young's workshops and classes and started teaching others about the benefits of fasting and detoxing which I still practice today.

Disclaimer: Juice fasting is not meant for everyone without supervision, particularly if you have pre-existing medical conditions. It is recommended you consult a professional for guidance.

SPIRITUAL BALANCE/ENERGY BALANCE

Whenever our lives feel like they are spiraling out of control, whether it is on a physical, mental or spiritual level, most will reconnect to their spiritual and religious roots. Whatever your spiritual practices or affiliation is, it reconnects you to the universal source of creation, something we feel is higher than ourselves. This connection allows you to soothe your soul and calm your mind. There are many forms of spiritual practice that can be used whether through prayer, meditation, scriptures, music, a religious community or communing in nature. This practice helps to ground us and connect us to all of creation and to ourselves.

In my quest to find *balance* I have used spiritual affirmations, biblical teachings, inspirational music, books, lectures and connection to like-minded spiritual partners/counselors who could assist me with gaining perspective and insight into what may be occurring in my life, world and affairs.

Prayer and meditation have assisted me and others around the world to connect with that inner spirit that is within all of us. The benefits also assist in better health and mental functions to center you and help with breathing and relaxing the mind and body which assist in better sleep habits and mental clarity during awake periods.

You cannot function and maintain balance if there is a disconnect with yourself.

Most alternative health practices incorporate some form of spiritual balance when addressing physical and mental dis-ease.

During my healing process I connected with a spiritual community, Christ Universal Temple in Chicago, that practiced spiritual/historical/metaphysical teachings under the teachings of Dr. Johnnie Coleman. It was new to me and allowed me to think differently about the mind/body/spirit connection; there is no separation and each part affects the other.

First, I learned about the power of positive thinking, the law of attraction and manifesting the things you desire including health and well-being. The concept of what you think, feel, believe and speak will manifest in your life. The principle of focusing more on what you desire and less on what you do not is the key to changing your thoughts, which will ultimately change your life. If you desire health, focus on perfect health and not on dis-ease so that your body can respond to the positive thoughts. If you desire prosperity, focus on abundance and not on the lack and so on. I started to take classes and practice these new principles and affirm positive thoughts, and my mental and spiritual mind started to positively affect my physical body.

It was at the time when the self-help era was booming, and there are still a host of concepts and ideologies that you can learn and incorporate in your daily life.

I met a metaphysician practitioner who was an expert on quantum transformational and spiritual approaches to healing who was also a licensed acupuncturist and trained from various countries in Reiki (energy work), oriental massage and acupressure. Dr. Deidre Burrell had her own practice, a local TV show called *Harmonious Vibrations* and held weekend holistic retreats for women. I attended multiple retreats and programs and had my first of several acupuncture treatments she provided to balance my "Chi" (life force energy or **vital life of a living being** in traditional Chinese philosophy, religion and medicine) and "Chakras" (each of the centers of spiritual power in the human body, usually considered to be seven in number).

She subsequently became my mentor and I worked with her for many years.

The power of the mind and its impact on our physical health conditions can not be underestimated. We are just starting to see in modern medicine the acknowledgment that our mental/emotional health is just as important as our physical health and that each affects the other. It is also equally important to provide the spiritual component as well as we are also starting to see more and more chaplains and ministerial/religious staff utilized in our healthcare institutions to assist patients in the healing process. Integrative medicine is being used in chronic care treatments as well as hospice end-of-life care. It is imperative in the comprehensive "whole person" model of care, now and in the future.

AROMATHERAPY—ESSENTIAL OILS

According to the National Center for Complementary and Integrative Health, "Aromatherapy is the use of essential oils from plants (flowers, herbs, or trees) as a complementary health approach. The essential oils are most often used by inhaling them or by applying a diluted form to the skin."[xii] Sometimes it's called essential oil therapy.

Verywell Health notes that "Essential oils are often used to ease stress, boost mood, relieve pain from headaches and migraines, get a better sleep, quell nausea, and even repel insects."[xiii]

According to Oils of the Bible, "essential oils are referenced in thirty-six out of thirty-nine books of the Old Testament and ten of the twenty-seven books of the New

Testament. They are mentioned more than 500 times in the Bible!"xiv

Precious oils were used to anoint and heal the sick throughout the Bible. The Three Wise Men, or Magi, brought essential oils as a gift to the Christ child. These oils have healing, therapeutic properties and were often used as medicine in biblical times.

There are many more oils listed in the Bible. Below are seven primary oils:

1. Cassia
2. Cypress
3. Frankincense
4. Myrrh
5. Roman Chamomile
6. Sandalwood
7. Spikenard

When I was trying to find ways to relax my mind and increase my restful sleep so that my body could repair, essential oils and aromatherapy were a helpful addition to my regular health regimen. Aromatherapy has assisted me and countless others in having better clarity and is a great accompaniment to my meditation practices.

The above areas of alternative/complementary health are not a complete list of all the variety of techniques and treatments that are available and utilized by millions around the world. They only represent the most popular ones that are becoming more familiar in Western society. These approaches are the ones that I have personally used myself and have over the years assisted others in their road to restore balance in certain areas of their life. Even though we have advanced tremendously in diagnostic testing, surgical procedures, drug therapy and other areas of treatments, certain age-old techniques never lose their significance and benefits.

My personal and professional belief is that we do not have to eliminate all the past practices and benefits that are more natural in their approach in place of our new modern advancements. We can do both and still create some form of balance in our healthcare system through integrative approaches that utilize the best of both approaches. It is something to be said about what our grandparents and great-grandparents practiced when access to healthcare was limited and not available to all citizens. African, Native American, European, Asian, South American, the Caribbean and Mexican countries all still use some form of natural, historical cultural practices where it relates to health on a regular basis with the exception of our Western culture in America on a large scale.

With the increase of chronic diseases and millions of people suffering with physical and mental dis-eases in this country, particularly people of color and the poor, we can by *choice* start to look at *all* options and follow the rest of the world and integrate some of the holistic treatments that have been available since the beginning of recorded time or by *force* as we continue to have some of the worst health outcomes as a developed country in the world.

JOURNALING

Journaling, or as some used to call it, writing in a diary, your thoughts and feelings down helps you to release pent-up emotions and racing thoughts. It is a practice that many have benefitted from to slow down and refocus the mind.

This regular practice has helped me throughout the years to express my feelings and set my intentions and goals. I started writing down my thoughts as well as incorporating a daily gratitude journal of the things I was grateful for so as to not focus on negative thoughts. I can look back at some of my journal entries and see how far I have come and the goals I have achieved and others that still need my attention.

University of Rochester Medical Center determined the benefits of journaling for mental health: "One of the ways to deal with any overwhelming emotion is to find a healthy way to express yourself...Journaling can help you manage anxiety, reduce stress and cope with depression."[xv]

Others have used ceremonial activities like writing down your negative thoughts and burning them or throwing them in an ocean. These are practices and activities that can clear your mind and spirit to balance your mental thoughts. Proverbs 23:7 (NKJV) says, "For as he thinks in his heart, so *is* he. 'Eat and drink!' he says to you, But his heart is not with you."[xvi]

Think good thoughts and your actions will follow.

*"When life knocks you down, try to land on your back.
Because if you can look up, you can get up."*

—Les Brown

.

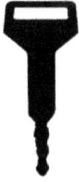

Key 4. (Re)boot

(After crash/stops working because of
malfunction/to start again)

Shantell is a fifty-one-year-old who has been a practicing pescatarian for over twenty-five years. She was raised under the current traditional American diet and made a decision in her late twenties to incorporate a healthier lifestyle. It was a gradual process: first, she eliminated certain foods (starting with pork, red meat, and then eventually chicken), eating only fish/seafood, then stopped consuming dairy products and processed sugars and doing occasional mini-fasts on juices, trying colonics, taking herbs/vitamins, using natural products, etc. She was so pleased by the way she felt and looked that she introduced her new healthy lifestyle to her family and friends and anyone who would listen and had very few, if any, health challenges over the years. Shantell was such a natural health enthusiast that she decided that holistic health was the only way and did not visit a traditional medical provider for twenty years other than during her pregnancies.

After turning fifty she started having problems with her gums and teeth but ignored them for a period of time. Once they became a chronic dental problem she visited her dentist who, to her surprise, found bone loss and was perplexed and referred her to a medical doctor who ran a battery of tests to realize she had an overactive thyroid (Hyperthyroidism), and calcium excess (which required an emergency infusion) due to a malfunctioning parathyroid which resulted in surgical *removal and follow-up treatments and medication to restore balance in her glandular system.*

During her healing process, Shantell didn't just focus on the physical dis-ease; she also wanted to understand and heal the spiritual and mental dis-ease and imbalance in her life. She realized that even when you attempt to do all the right things to create a healthy life, it requires all three areas to be whole and healthy. She was forced to also focus on herself (mental and spirit) to get to the root of her imbalance and dis-ease. It required authentic truth about areas of family wounds and not speaking her truths and emotional pain (holistically the throat represents swallowed anger, an inability to speak up for one's self). She is now working on creating balance in all areas of her life and becoming whole again.

This is a perfect example of how the body works as a whole and not in separate organs/systems. Dental health is also an indication of your physical health. When you have inflammation in your gums or bone loss it is an indication of the same conditions in the whole body. There is no separation between the whole body, mind and spirit.

Another important lesson from Shantell's experience is that practicing a holistic lifestyle (or some call it alternative health practices) still requires you to have an integrative approach and that includes medical screenings to determine if there are any imbalances or deficiencies that may need to be addressed. Then you can make an informed decision on what would be the best approach or treatments to resolve any health issues. In my opinion and experience, using the best of both approaches can assist in creating balance in the healing process.

Rebooting after a crash or burn out requires at times in life for us to start again. Just like a computer may be working fine and out of nowhere (we think) it just crashes and stops working even though we may have gotten warnings and systems moving slower than normal, we continue to just keep working without evaluation and maintenance.

We believe we did a great job of keeping up the maintenance to keep it running smoothly and no matter how much and how long we used or abused it, it will continue to work. All the while never deleting or upgrading to free up space, instead we just keep downloading too many files that may have a virus and suddenly, unexpectedly it crashes and stops working.

It is the same with our mind, body and spirit. We believe we are balancing our life, (eating healthy foods, taking supplements, exercising, resting and having a spiritual practice), but we are also required to purge the old mental and emotional stuff before adding new stuff (detox the body and spirit). Many holistic practitioners advocate to detox the old junk rather than just build the body or you will just build on a weak foundation. It requires *you* to get real with yourself. What's still lingering in your heart? What haven't you let go of? What toxic thoughts or beliefs are polluting your mind and ultimately your body? What resentments may you still be holding on to?

If you don't *choose* to deal with past wounds, hurts and resentments, they may show up in the present as dis-ease where you are *forced* to address it.

We're taught in the holistic health field that every physical dis-ease has an emotional and mental equivalent that is the root cause. For example, having unforgiveness and resentment is like drinking poison and thinking you're hurting the other person. They've moved on, but you haven't. As a result, your pressure is elevated or you're otherwise negatively physically affected.

When you're doing a full detox holistically, you're purging your body of toxins with a detox and incorporating healthy habits but you're also purging your mind from toxic thoughts through forgiveness activities, affirmations and your meditations to see what comes up when you're "quiet and still" and who still triggers emotions in you. Sometimes you think you're over something until you're around a particular someone or thoughts keep coming up years later. When it still controls your thoughts, it will eventually control your body. There is a saying: "Energy flows where attention goes," good, bad or indifferent. You can create healing with your thoughts/emotions but you also can create toxicity in your body when you hold on to low-vibrating emotions.

After a physical challenge, *you* can reboot by addressing not just the symptoms of the physical dis-ease or dis-comfort but also what mentally or spiritually may be causing this to show up in your life.

You will never get high blood pressure or any health conditions under control if you're still dealing with anger, bitterness, resentment and unforgiveness. You can eat healthy all day long, exercise daily and still have health challenges if you do not release and purge yourself of those toxic thoughts and emotions. You have to look at everything from a physical, emotional and spiritual standpoint.

During my own personal healing journey, I had to restart multiple times to create balance. Not only trying many of the holistic practices and treatments I discussed in the previous chapters to create hormonal balance, but also, I was *forced* to get serious on my spiritual journey to fully understand the mind-body-spirit connection. I knew that starting those holistic practices of taking vitamins, doing occasional juice fasts/detoxing, yoga and meditation was one part, but I was also required to connect my body with my spirit and to reboot and reprogram my mental thoughts towards healing and not dis-ease and that is when I started to see results in my life and have been teaching others since that time. As my spiritual teacher Johnnie Coleman taught and I found out to be true of the universal principles: "It works, if you work it!"

*"Wisdom **is** the principal thing; **Therefore** get wisdom.
And in all your getting, get understanding."*

—Proverbs 4:7 (NKJV)[xvii]

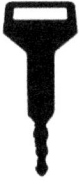

Key 5. (Re)adjust

(Make slight changes until you get it right)

When you are *forced* to *slow down* in life you are required to readjust your life, sometimes in a dramatic way that is out of your control. You will find that readjusting will require you to keep making changes until your new way of living becomes achievable and comfortable for you. You may find that after you think you have it figured out then something else requires you to make adjustments again until you know what works for you. We attempt to model the same approach for everyone and it just doesn't work for the masses of people, which creates health disparities and inequities. So not only do we have to readjust as individuals, but also in our approach as a collective whole in order to see a shift in our outcomes.

There is not a one-size-fits-all approach to anything and we have to remember we are all unique, unrepeatable, individualized expressions of God. As the saying goes, everything doesn't work for everybody. Just like snowflakes, we are created the same but are not all the same. That doesn't mean the universal principles do not work; you just have to find out which ones will work for *you*! It requires you to understand how you function, to tune into your body and spirit so you can identify and know when it is out of alignment and balance. And no one can do that for you but *you*. Others, whether medical, psychological or spiritual professionals, are only partners to assist you with the healing process.

It is surprising to me as a health professional how little I knew about my own body's needs until I was *forced* to, and how many people I come across, young, old, rich, poor, educated and uneducated, who do not fully understand their bodies, how they work and what they require to create a balanced state. We seek out many things outside ourselves (material, physical appearance, etc.) but we spend very little time educating ourselves on self-care and understanding the physical temple that houses our spirit.

Many adults still do not understand the basic operations of our organs and body systems and how they all work together which we should have mastered in school. And we definitely did not learn how our bodies are connected to the universal earthly body. In ancient and early civilizations, we understood how the micro (humans) and the macro (universe) is all connected, how our menstrual cycles are related to the moon cycles and that of the earth—our energy and emotional cycles as well. At one point in time, our ancestors planned when to conceive based on the earthly cycle in conjunction with the feminine cycle, similar to the animal kingdom. They planted their foods on a cycle so that the earth would have time to replenish, etc.

We were not taught that there is an energy to everything in the universe that operates on a certain frequency. I later learned on my journey that everything in the universe is energetic. We all vibrate at a different frequency. That is why we can feel the vibration of others' energy just by being in their presence and in our thoughts where you can feel someone thinking about you and then suddenly, they contact you.

We were not taught that our foods also have energy and frequency. There is a difference between live foods versus dead foods. Live foods—fruits and vegetables—have a higher vibration and give more energy, whereas dead foods (chips, over-cooked, processed and boxed foods) weigh you down and deplete your energy to the point where you want to go to sleep.

I wasn't taught that in the past. We weren't taught the therapeutic benefits of the sun and the Vitamin D connection and the benefits of natural light and fresh air for our bodies. In our current modern lifestyles, we are in our homes and offices more with artificial lighting all day and now they're coming up with different types of light bulbs to try to reduce the electromagnetic rays and to try to mimic natural light. Because we are indoors more often, salt lamps and diffusers are now popular to help purify the air. So, we're trying to get back to some sources of natural connection to the earth. But unfortunately, in this new progressive society, it can be difficult to do on a daily basis. You have to really make some effort. We're going to have to incorporate some of the things that have been tried and true, but we don't have to throw away all of our science and innovation to get back to some basic practices. We're just going to have to balance it out and use wisdom from the past because all of the new modern technological advancements are not the healthiest for us. And we will have to readjust back to some of the approaches from the past. We're one of the most advanced countries in this world, but yet we still are suffering due to lack of knowledge, understanding or unwillingness.

My experience with others has shown that we are still resistant to some basic concepts and are *forced* many times to readjust. When we are *forced* to do anything, we will try with urgency to attempt to get fast results and get discouraged when the outcome does not manifest in the instantaneous time frame we expect based on lack of attention on our part when we had flashing lights and signals warning us to make a *choice* to make adjustments. Once we realize we are *forced* to readjust our behavior or thinking, then it may shock us into action. In our modern-day medical approach, more emphasis is on treating versus prevention. Unfortunately, when we don't understand or respond to the signs, then the treatment approach may require an aggressive solution to get back to balance.

*Karen was in her thirties and loved to live life to the fullest. She had a fun, outgoing personality and had a hot, spicy life and she enjoyed her foods the same way. She started with mild digestive problems which led to acid reflux occasionally when she ate her hot, spicy foods. She enjoyed hot sauce on everything including her snacks. It became chronic and eventually she woke up with stomach pain, vomiting and could not even keep down liquids. She was rushed to the hospital and found out her stomach lining was so corroded that the doctors described it as if someone had poured gasoline down her throat and inflamed her stomach. She was put on a high dose of morphine for pain and one of the strongest antibiotics to help heal the ulcerated stomach lining which cost about $300 out of pocket. She was bedridden and couldn't afford the prescription. She then by **force** and severe pain was willing to try a twenty-one-day detox and liquid juice fast. Her stomach lining healed slowly and she was eventually able to resume eating regular foods. She tried to maintain a healthy lifestyle but returned back to her old conditioned habits and by forty she had large gallstones and was rushed to an emergency gall bladder removal surgery in the middle of the night, and at this point she did not have a **choice**.*

She has since recovered and gotten serious with her health, has lost a significant amount of weight, exercises daily and is now committed to living a healthy, balanced life.

Even though Karen's journey required multiple readjustments, and she was *forced* to make multiple attempts, she continued until she found a process that worked for her that she could maintain and that she could incorporate into her everyday lifestyle.

We cannot continue with the current American healthcare model that offers a one-size-fits-all approach to healthcare. Even in the natural health industry we cannot expect everyone to be able to readjust their way of living their entire life and become a health enthusiast overnight. That is not sustainable, affordable or practical for the average person. So many times, instead of taking small steps to better health many *choose* to not do anything because they feel defeated when they do not accomplish goals that are not a good fit for them.

When working with myself and others, I alter it in a way that people can digest it. As I once heard in a sermon, "You can't give a baby meat who doesn't have teeth. You have to start them on baby food and slowly build them up to meat." Similarly, you can't just start someone on a thirty-day liquid fast. You have to gradually get it to where they can digest the information and lifestyle and keep building on it, so it'll be something they can incorporate. Similar to Karen, when I was *forced* to, I jumped right in and did what I needed to feel better including a thirty-day liquid fast, but with others it can be modified with a gradual approach for them. Instead of cutting out meat and dairy for thirty days, we start out with meatless Mondays. Even my soul food-loving friends and family started to turn around after seeing the journey I was on and the results I was experiencing. One friend gave up pork and red meat indefinitely. My mom replaced red meat with turkey. And others started doing a bi-annual detox with me to purge the body of toxins to give their body's time to rejuvenate and restore.

The all-or-nothing mentality, I believe, is a huge turn off for many looking at the holistic industry. There's middle ground and plenty of it. If you take simple steps, small steps can lead to bigger steps. So, it's a disadvantage to believe that if you can't do the whole thing then you can't do it at all. With each goal you achieve, it'll give you more confidence and ability to go further with it.

Once I started using this strategy, I observed less resistance with family, friends and clients. They were more willing to try some recommendations even if they didn't feel confident that they could maintain everything. Last year, for instance, I facilitated a detox with ten other women. I explained that many detoxes involve raw fasting, but that we were going to do a modified version with vegan foods similar to Daniel's Fast (in Christian practices during Lenten season) where you just try to eat whole foods. Let's start with 60/40. You eat 60 percent raw and 40 percent cooked. They were all successful; but had I approached them with all raw or straight juice, most would not have successfully completed their first time.

One of the traditional public health models that was taught in my graduate school program helps you to understand the different stages you may go through when incorporating new behaviors or lifestyles when you start to readjust your life, and that is the "5 Primary Stages of Behavior Change" as outlined in the book *Changing for Good*:[xviii]

5 STAGES OF BEHAVIOR CHANGE MODEL

1. **Precontemplation**: People in this stage don't want to make any change to their habits and don't recognize that they have any problems/issues.
2. **Contemplation**: Knowing you need to make changes and thinking about what you may need to do.
3. **Preparation**: Preparing for the changes or new behaviors.
4. **Action**: Actively working on the changes.
5. **Maintenance**: Making the changes a permanent part of your life.

Many times, you will go through these steps multiple times before it becomes a habit or a lifestyle. Since the body's cells regenerate approximately every twenty-one to twenty-seven days, it is a common recommendation that you incorporate any health practice for at least twenty-one days so that it can become a permanent practice and have long standing benefits.

The lesson: readjust when necessary and repeat!

"Heal yourself first. The rest will come later!"

—Unknown

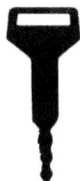

Key 6. (Re)start

(A new beginning/to resume after interruption)

New beginnings are sometimes *Scary*! When you restart anything in life after an interruption you are initially nervous, afraid and uncertain about the change. Whether it is a health crisis, relationship breakup, career change, children, etc., change and starting over can be difficult. You are moving into uncharted territory and you can become fearful that nothing will ever be the same. And just maybe that may be a good thing.

Of course, with any restart or change in your life, guilt will rear its ugly head. You start thinking it is selfish to put yourself first, or to give up the expectations that others have for you but may be slowly killing you (physically and mentally). You tell yourself "but I have too much to do" or "too many people are depending on me to focus on myself" or "I cannot afford to give up that stressful job" or a million and one other obligations we continue to commit to even though we have enough on our plate.

For women, but also for men, the above quotes create a lot of mixed emotions. Putting yourself first just doesn't sit well with people when there are so many people who need help or when you have a multitude of responsibilities. But at what cost are you willing to put everything and everybody first and risk your own life? And I state again the saying, put your own oxygen mask on first before helping others.

Henrietta was a giver her entire life. At a young age she was responsible for all her younger brothers and sisters and even younger extended family. She became a mother figure before she was even a mother. Once she became a mother at a young age, she was still expected by her family to take care of everyone including the elders in the family without rarely ever having a life for herself or fulfilling any of her childhood dreams. This continued her entire adult life and, in her fifties, she started to have health challenges but kept them secret because she wasn't accustomed to focusing on herself and didn't know how to ask for help for herself, only how to give help to others. In her silence, her health slowly became worse and her family didn't notice because she was always the strong one. One day she sprained her knee and went to the doctor's only after she could barely walk and found out at that appointment that her heart was having arrythmias at 150 to 160 beats a minute (normal is under one hundred) and the doctor wondered how she was still able to function. It's like you are constantly running a race while sitting in place. They immediately rushed her to the hospital and after numerous tests, it was found her heart was only functioning at 30 percent (which is almost disabled) and the doctors were baffled that she never had symptoms or was still functioning through the day. Her heart had to be electrically shocked back into rhythm restart in order for her heart muscle to rest and rebuild. After *multiple hospital stays, procedures, defibrillator and permanent medications Henrietta is finally managing her condition and has been **forced** to pay attention to herself and the needs of her body.*

When we are so focused on others, we can miss the subtle symptoms and signs that our body is trying to tell us that it is out of balance until it has to scream to get our attention.

This was the dilemma I found myself in when I was *forced* to pause. I kept thinking, "You have a husband, baby and a preschooler, a career you don't want to interrupt again and multiple financial responsibilities." Your mind is saying, how can you afford to pause and restart? But my body said, how can you afford not to? It requires courage and conviction to put yourself first and not worry about what others may think, feel or say about it. It also requires unwavering commitment to yourself to convince yourself that it is in the best interest of everyone if you show up in the world your best, whole, balanced self. As I always tell others now, you can only give from the overflow and you cannot pour out from an empty vessel. The job, relationship, money and friends will all hopefully still be there once you are whole. And if not, as the saying goes, they were not supposed to be there any longer and served their purpose in your life.

When I was able to slow down and focus on myself, still having obligations but letting go of anything that interfered with the healing process (the titles, career for a moment, salary, volunteer work, etc.), I learned a lot about myself and what I needed to shift in my life. When I was able to get still, I then found that my symptoms as described in the earlier chapter were a result of hormonal imbalance, perimenopause (even though I was told multiple times I was too young) and adrenal fatigue (due to stress and the common "disease to please" syndrome).

I was blessed to be able to take the time to discover through trial and error and consulting with various holistic practitioners what I needed to do, as mentioned in the previous chapters, to bring wellness back into my life, mind, body and spirit. This time to focus on myself literally restarted and changed my life and placed me on my personal journey to authentic truth, spiritual enlightenment and wholistic balance.

When I tried to only focus on the physical symptoms, I didn't have the full benefits. I then had to seek out spiritual practices and also change my mental thought patterns to fully start to have balance in my life.

Now working with others, I find that there is a hesitation for many to put themselves first, similar to Henrietta and my past self and to balance out the competing priorities in their lives until they are *forced* to and have very few options. They have many excuses and reasons why they will focus on themselves at some later date or pre-determined time when everything else is in place, but unfortunately, I have witnessed too often that some never get the chance until it's too late or not at all.

So my question to you is, what's preventing you from taking care of yourself first?

"I have come to believe that caring for myself is not self-indulgent.

Caring for myself is an act of survival."

—Audre Lorde

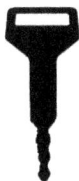

Key 7. (Re)new

(After a pause/more energy and
strength/to restore to existence/ the act
or process of becoming spiritually new)

The journey to wholeness and balance is not a straight path. It can have many twists and turns and stumbles and failures along the way. Through trial and error, you find what works for *you* and what does not. You learn to experiment with what you can sustain on a regular basis and what may be a one-time attempt, and of course you can spend a lot of time and money (literally pay now or pay later) before you finally find the keys to be renewed! Which will look different for each person, as we are made the same but not all the same.

As stated before, I have personally tried many methods, products, practices, etc. before I found a personalized program that worked for me. I read an exhaustive amount of self-help books, attended many classes, conferences and lectures that focused on the mind, body and spirit. As one of my favorite authors, the late Wayne Dyer stated, I was "Open to everything and attached to nothing." I was willing to try and incorporate whatever I could find to feel renewed again.

I was open to learning new things and letting go of old habits, beliefs and family customs passed down that no longer served me (like eating meat at every meal or seasoning all my vegetables with pork) which prevented me from feeling my best self. I fully understood that self-care was an act of survival and not selfish as we are taught when we decide to focus on our own well-being.

Once I identified that I ultimately had a hormonal imbalance and was just doing too much (a typical modern-day woman trait), I was able through the help of programs to incorporate nutritional supplements, certain whole foods and daily spiritual and holistic practices and started changing my thoughts and some behaviors; and then I was finally able to feel balanced and renewed again.

Once I realized the power of my thoughts and started understanding and believing the healing power of every cell, visualizing and affirming that my body and mind was perfect, whole and complete, I started to also experience the mental and spiritual breakthrough and my physical improvement followed. I had to address my limiting beliefs and societal conditioning first. I didn't grow up knowing our bodies can regenerate in the right environment given the right tools. And the most important part is that healing is possible, just by the renewing of your mind. That was the biggest revelation.

That was over fifteen years ago and I have been able to maintain many of the practices and benefits I discovered even though I am not perfect or consistent in all areas; I know the process and the practices work and totally changed the direction of my life. It took about two years before I felt renewed to be able to go back into my career and all the things I'd tried to do before but couldn't, but now with balance. I actually accomplish even more now and juggle more responsibilities than before as I am now aware of when I am out of alignment and take those periods of pause by *choice* to restore and renew. I fully understand and appreciate that self-care is an act of survival and it is imperative that we practice it daily.

Renewal is a verb (an action word not just a noun). It is a continuous process and doesn't stop once you overcome a crisis or start to feel better. Just the fact that the blood cells have a life span of about 120 days and we receive new cells for our organs every twelve months and no cell is older than seven years shows that we were wonderfully and intelligently made to renew continuously. And just as our body's cells die off and renew, so should our minds and spirits. Dr. Christiane Northup, a pioneer in women's health, states about ageless women that "getting older is inevitable; aging is optional,"[xix] and that is based on the renewal process of the mind, body and spirit.

Surprisingly, none of this information is new information and many of these renewing practices have been used around the world since the beginning of time across many nationalities and cultures; but unfortunately, in American progressive society we are not taught in most of our families the tools and practices to maintain health and balance, and the cultural customs of our ancestors are considered outdated and not used by most individuals due to so-called progress and advancements. We are no longer in-tune with the physical body let alone the earthly body which has always been connected to us.

Do *you* know when you're out of alignment, and do you listen to those signs and messages? Or do you just distract yourself with busyness and numerous activities while you ignore signs that you need to *slow down*?

The question we now have to ask today in our fast-paced society is, do we have to do away with customs and practices that have worked since the beginning of the universe and humankind in place of advancement and technology, or is there room for both in our so-called advanced world? I personally believe that we can benefit from both by going back to some basics from the past and incorporate the present advancements.

If not, at what cost do we pay for our physical, mental and spiritual health?

With the rapid increase in dis-ease in our advanced societies, now more than ever it is time to be mindful and pay attention inwardly and outwardly to the signals to *slow down* by *choice* when necessary or *lay down* by *force*!

The choice is ultimately within and it's ours to decide. I pray we *choose* to listen and trust our internal GPS (God's Protective System) that navigates and directs us all!

"Sometimes you have to let go of the picture of what you thought life would be like and learn to find joy in the story you are actually living."

—Rachel Martin

CLOSING

2020 Universal Slow Down
(Covid-19 Quarantine)

Slow Down by Choice or Lay Down by Force started as my personal journey and the journey of my clients back to wholeness and balance by being *forced* to *slow down* in various periods of our individual lives.

And then entered 2020, the year of the coronavirus (COVID-19) and a universal *slow down* (quarantine) on Earth. 2020 is also in numerology (the science of numbers) a four year (two plus zero plus two plus zero) which represents upheaval, hard work, restriction and building new foundations/systems after dismantling outdated systems. How timely and prophetic.

This year's changes and challenges, which we have never experienced in our generation, still should not come as a total surprise if we think deeply on the theme of this writing; we have had signs for many years personally and universally to *slow down* by *choice* and have ultimately (some say unexpectedly although I don't believe in accidents, just the universe's way of getting our attention) been *forced* through a universal quarantine to combat the spread of COVID-19. It has been a devastating and humbling experience in every country on the planet and has affected all our lives. So, what lessons have we learned from this pandemic and *forced* Quarantine?

In every experience there is a lesson, no matter how unnerving or tragic, to teach us how to use the experience as a catalyst for something even greater in our lives. When attempting to understand or make sense of any perceived negative situation or circumstance, it is best for our mental, physical and spiritual health after the initial shock and emotional natural responses to start to analyze what the positive aspects are that can assist us in growing through the challenges.

Focus when you can on what you desire to happen and not on the appearance of the problem/circumstance that has currently shown up in your life. By focusing on what you desire and not what you don't, you set an intention for yourself to start to creatively think and act on a process of how to work through to manifest those desires.

I and others have identified and discovered that there have been some benefits to this *forced* quarantine experience even though it has been as equally devastating and disruptive in many of our lives and in the world.

For example, an article from News Gram[xx] stated that there have been some earthly benefits to the Lockdown of 2020: "The COVID-19 lockdowns globally have not only made air breathable or rivers clean but have also resulted in the way our Earth moves, as researchers now report a drop in seismic noise (the hum of vibrations in the planet's crust) because transport networks, real estate and other human activities have been shut down." This means that the planet itself is moving a little less, and based on a journal article in *Nature*, it "could allow detectors to spot smaller earthquakes and boost efforts to monitor volcanic activity and other seismic events."[xxi]

I stated in earlier chapters that everything on the planet has an energetic vibration/frequency. We basically can now listen to the vibrational sounds and warnings of the Universe and how they connect to us physically, mentally and spiritually. Isn't that what we all say we have experienced in Quarantine? We can now hear our inner body's signals, thoughts/desires/goals, and each other as we have been *forced* to *slow down* and hear the messages and lessons that we could not hear in all our busyness and activity while in constant motion.

Psalms 46:10 (NIV) reminds us, *"He says, 'Be still, and know that I am God; I will be exalted among the nations, I will be exalted in the earth.'"*[xxii]

Is this the reason for the "Universal Slow Down"? So we can get in alignment and in-tune to renew the earth and our own individual lives, as many of us have abused both for many years?

I have heard many say during this quarantine and pandemic experience that it has allowed themselves to slow down and strengthen their spiritual practices, bond with their families, commune with nature, focus on their physical health, let their voices be heard about injustices and inequality in various forms and work as a universal community (frontline essential workers) to assist others during this difficult time.

Individually and collectively, as we move beyond this experience and used this *forced* time to go to our own individual sacred space within where all answers are revealed, prayerfully we will have shifted in our thinking and ways of living and we will have listened and learned the lessons that God will have us to learn by our own *choice* so that equity and balance will permeate the earth and all its inhabitants for many, many years. During these challenging times, this song represents for me that sacred space where all healing and connection to our higher selves takes place that we all have been *forced* to *slow down* and experience during this time.

"Sacred Space" by India.Arie

"Where I go to be moved, where I go to be still, your love makes me new, in your presence I heal.

You are my favorite place, you are my sacred space, yes you are, yes you are, yes you are!"

GLOSSARY

Chakras. Seven energy centers of spiritual power in the human body.

Chi. Life force energy or **vital life of a living being** in traditional Chinese philosophy, religion and medicine.

Dead foods. Refined, highly processed, not in its natural state with little nutritional value.

Dis-ease. Not in its normal state, lack of ease, not functioning properly, a body working outside of the law of life.

Live foods. Foods as close to their original, natural form (plants, fruits, vegetables).

Re. Prefix. Represents going backward, repetition, withdrawal.

SAD. Stands for Standard American Diet void of vitamins, minerals, nutrients, fiber etc.

Seven. Represents spiritual perfection, sacredness, completeness, inner wisdom, introspection, rest.

Wholistic. An alternate spelling of "Holistic" to represent the wholeness within Man/Woman achieved through merging Mind/Body/Spirit.

Journal

What ways do you create balance
in your daily life?

Mentally

Mentally

Mentally

Mentally

_____

_____

_____

_____

_____

_____

_____

_____

_____

_____

_____

_____

_____

_____

_____

_____

_____

_____

Physically

_____

_____

_____

_____

_____

_____

_____

_____

_____

_____

_____

_____

_____

_____

_____

_____

_____

_____

Physically

Physically

_____

_____

_____

_____

_____

_____

_____

_____

_____

_____

_____

_____

_____

_____

_____

_____

_____

_____

_____

Physically

_____

_____

_____

_____

_____

_____

_____

_____

_____

_____

_____

_____

_____

_____

_____

_____

_____

_____

_____

_____

Spiritually

_____

_____

_____

_____

_____

_____

_____

_____

_____

_____

_____

_____

_____

_____

_____

_____

_____

_____

_____

_____

_____

Spiritually

_____

_____

_____

_____

_____

_____

_____

_____

_____

_____

_____

_____

_____

_____

_____

_____

_____

_____

_____

Spiritually

Spiritually

NOTES

All chapter beginning definitions are from Hornblower, Simon, Antony Spawforth, and Esther Eidinow. The Oxford Classical Dictionary. Oxford: Oxford University Press, 2012.

Key 2

i.   Suni, Eric. "Insomnia – Symptoms, Types, Causes, and More." SleepFoundation. OneCare Media, LLC., September 4, 2020. http://www.sleepfoundation.org/insomnia.

ii.   Mayo Clinic Staff. "Insomnia." Mayo Clinic. Mayo Foundation for Medical Education and Research, October 15, 2016. http://www.mayoclinic.org/diseases-conditions/insomnia/symptoms-causes/syc-20355167.

iii. Wilson, James L. "What Is Hypoadrenia and Adrenal Fatigue." In Adrenal Fatigue: the 21st Century Stress Syndrome, 7–9. Petaluma, CA: Smart Publications, 2017.

iv.   Holy Bible: New International Version. Grand Rapids, MI: Zondervan, 2019.

Key 3

v.   Definitions, Meanings, Synonyms, and Grammar by Oxford Dictionary on Lexico.com. (2020). Retrieved November 07, 2020, from http://www.lexico.com/.

vi.   Byrne, Rhonda. The Secret. New York, NY: Atria Books, 2018.

vii.   Ratini, Melinda. "Holistic Medicine: What It Is, Treatments, Philosophy, and More." WebMD. WedbMD LLC., March 18, 2020. https://www.web-md.com/balance/guide/what-is-holistic-medicine.

viii.   Shiel, MD, W. C. "Definition of Oriengtal Medicine (Traditional)." MedicineNet. MedicineNet, Inc. December 27, 2018. https://www.medicinenet.com/oriental_medicine_traditional/definition.htm.

ix.   Holy Bible: New International Version. Grand Rapids, MI, MI: Zondervan, 2019.

x.   Holy Bible: New International Version. Grand Rapids, MI, MI: Zondervan, 2019.

xi.   Dolittle, Dr. "Fasting as a Survival Strategy in Animals." ScienceBlogs. Science 2.0, September 27, 2017. https://scienceblogs.com/lifelines/2017/09/28/fasting-as-a-survival-strategy-in-animals.

xii.   "Aromatherapy." National Center for Complementary and Integrative Health. U.S. Department of Health and Human Services. January 2020. https://www.nccih.nih.gov/ health/aromatherapy.

xiii.   Wong, Cathy. "An Overview of Essential Oils." Edited by Meredith Bull. Verywell Health. About, Inc. (Dotdash), April 20, 2020. https://www.verywell-health.com/ what-are-essential-oils-88807.

xiv.   Robinson, Tracy. "Essential Oils of the Bible." Essential Homestead (blog), May 17, 2018.

www.essentailhomestead.com/essential-oils-bible
-essential-homestead/.

xv.   Watson, L Renee, Marianne Fraser, and Paul Ballas, eds. "Journaling for Mental Health," 2020. http://www.urmc.rochester.edu/.

xvi.   Holy Bible: The New King James Version, Containing the Old and New Testaments. Nashville, TN: T. Nelson, 1982.

Key 4
xvii. Holy Bible: the New King James Version, Containing the Old and New Testaments. Nashville, TN: T. Nelson, 1982.

Key 5
xviii. Prochaska, James O., John C. Norcross, and Carlo C. DiClemente. Changing for Good. New York, NY: Avon books, 1995.

Key 7
xix.   Northrup, Christiane. Goddesses Never Age: The Secret Prescription for Radiance, Vitality, and Well-Being. Carlsbad, CA: Hay House, 2016.

CLOSING
xx.   "The Positive Effect of Covid-19 Lockdown on Earth." NewsGram, April 5, 2020. www-newsgram.com/positive-effect-covid-19-lockdown-earth/.

xxi. Gibney, Elizabeth. "Coronavirus Lockdowns Have Changed the Way Earth Moves." Nature 580 (March 31, 2020): 176–77. https://doi.org/10.1038/d41586-020-00227-w.

xxii. Holy Bible: New International Version. Grand Rapids, MI, MI: Zondervan, 2019.

About the Author

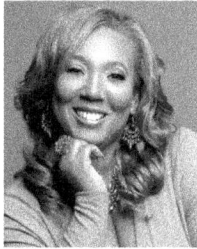

Trina Pitts-Khalfani's mission is to empower individuals to take control of their health through natural alternatives. She established Wholistic Balance, LLC, to educate clients on how to incorporate natural health practices into their daily lives.

Trina earned a B.S. in business administration from Morgan State University, an M.Ed in public health education from Penn State University, and then became a certified health education specialist and later a certified natural health professional. In 2011, she graduated with an ND as a naturopathic practitioner from Trinity School of Natural Health and became a board-certified naturopathic practitioner. Two years later, she was awarded a High Achievement Award by the American Naturopathic Medical Certification Board.

Trina currently resides in her home city of Harrisburg, Pennsylvania. She is passionate about community service and speaking on various public health and self-improvement topics. When she isn't working, Trina enjoys traveling and spending time with her two brilliant daughters.

To connect, visit Wholisticbalance.net email her at
Wholistic.balancelife@gmail.com

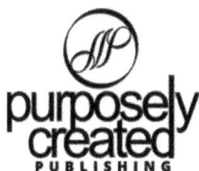

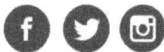